The Ultimate Dash Book for Be

Enjoy a Wide Selection of Super Af... Diet

Lola Rogers

Table of contents

Pomegranate and Peaches Avocado Toast

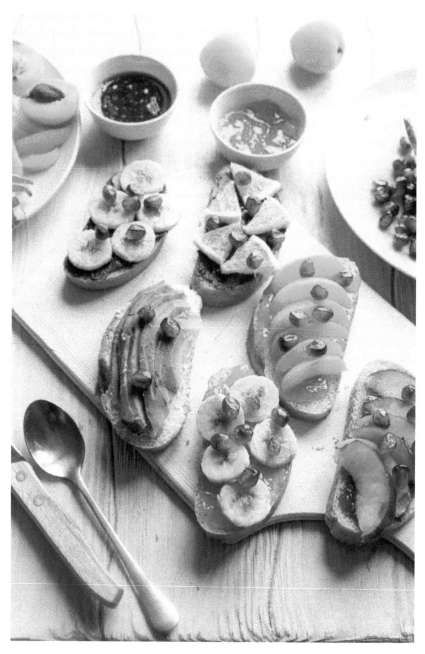

Ingredients

- one slice whole-grain bread
- 1/2 avocado
- 1 tbsp ricotta
- Pomegranate seeds, a small amount like one handful
- Drizzle honey

Directions

1. Toast the entire grain bread within the oven or toaster.

2. Spread avocado onto the toast, as smooth or coarse as you favor .

3. Spread a dollop of ricotta across the avocado.

4. Drizzle a piece of honey over the avocado mixture.

5. Sprinkle pomegranate seeds on top and luxuriate in .

Breakfast in a Jar

Ingredients

- 1/4 cup of oatmeal
- 3/4 cup of kefir
- 1 tbsp of chia seeds
- 2 tbsp of raisins
- 1 tbsp of unsweetened coconut flakes

Instructions

Make Layers of elements during a 16-ounce Mason jar , close the lid and

refrigerate overnight.

When it's able to eat, remove the jar from the fridge and provides it a fast stir.

Avocado Egg Cups

Ingredients

- Two avocados, ripe
- 1/4 tsp coarse salt
- 1/4 tsp pepper
- 1/2 tsp olive oil
- Four medium eggs
- 1 tbsp grated cheese, such as Parmesan, cheddar, or Swiss
- Assorted toppings: herbs, scallions, salsa, diced tomato, crumbled bacon, Sriracha, paprika, crumbled feta

Directions

1.   Heat oven to 375°F. Halve avocados lengthwise and pit. Cut a thin slice from bottom of every avocado half so that it sits level. Where Hell was, scoop out only enough of the flesh (about ½ tbsp) to form room for an egg.

2.   Place avocados on a foil-lined rimmed baking sheet. Season each with salt and pepper, and rub with vegetable oil .

3.   Crack an egg into each cavity (some of the albumen will run over the side, but don't be concerned about it). Sprinkle with cheese, if using. Cover loosely with foil.

4.   Bake almost 20 to 25 min, or until eggs are set to your liking. Sprinkle with toppings.

Sugar Break Apple and Peanut Butter Oatmeal

Ingredients

- 1 cup steel-cut oats
- Three medium-large Granny Smith apples, cored and sliced into 1-2" chunks
- A swirl of peanut butter
- pinch ground cinnamon
- 1 tbsp butter (optional)
- 4 cups of water
- pinch salt

Directions

Cook the oats till they reach the specified texture and creaminess.

Cut apples, toss them into the oats, and stir.

Then add spread into it and stir until melted and spread throughout.

Top with a touch of cinnamon and butter (optional) and enjoy!

Nutrient Calories: 453

Sweet Potato Toast

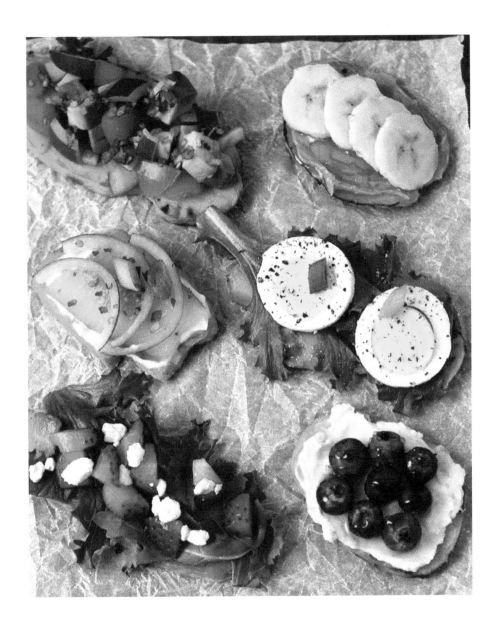

Ingredients

- One potato (sweet)

Instructions

1.   Divide the sweet potato into 1/4-inch slices and pop into the toaster.

2.   Top with anything you select . Popular combinations include spread with fruit, avocado, hummus, eggs,cheese, and tuna fish salad .

Nutrient Calories: 112

Italian Pasta Salad with Tomatoes and Artichoke Hearts

SmartPoints value: Green plan - 5SP, Blue plan - 5SP, Purple plan - 5SP

Total Time: 28 min, Prep time: 18 min, Cooking time: 10 min, Serves: 6

Nutritional value: Calories - 296.2, Carbs - 47.3g Fat - 8.2g, Protein - 8.7g

The best time to make this pasta salad is at the height of summer when fresh tomatoes are at their glorious, unrivalled peak. Make sure you use the ripest, juiciest tomatoes you can find. Tomato juices will add a delicious flavour to the dressing.

The chopped artichoke hearts will add a briny taste to every bite. Cellentani pasta is the macaroni formed into a spiral shape, also known as cavatappi. If you can't find that variety, feel free to use whatever type you can get, although short kinds of pasta like penne, rotini, and macaroni would work best. Turn this into a meal by adding some grilled or sautéed chicken or shrimp.

Ingredients

- Tomato(es) (fresh) - 1 pound(s), ripe beefsteak or Campari, chopped (3 cups)

- Bell pepper(s) (uncooked) - 2 item(s), small, yellow and orange, diced (1 ½ cups)

- Artichoke hearts without oil (canned) - 14 oz, drained, roughly chopped

- Basil (torn or coarsely chopped) - 1 cup(s)

- Red wine vinegar - 2 Tbsp

- Olive oil (extra virgin) - 2 Tbsp

- Table salt - ½ tsp, with extra for cooking pasta

- Black pepper - ½ tsp, freshly ground

- Garlic powder - ¼ tsp, or more to taste

- Pasta (uncooked) - 6 oz, cellentani recommended (2 cups)

- Parmesan cheese (shredded) - ⅓ cup(s), or shaved, divided

Instructions

1. Combine artichoke hearts, basil, tomatoes, peppers, vinegar, oil, salt, pepper, and garlic powder in a large bowl, then toss to coat. Allow the pasta to stand while cooking, occasionally tossing.

2. Boil a pot of well-salted water and cook the pasta according to package directions. Drain and rinse it with cold water, then drain again.

3. Add the pasta to the bowl with tomato mixture and toss to coat. Add all but two Tbsp Parmesan and toss again.

4. Serve the pasta salad with the remaining cheese sprinkled over to the top.

Tofu-veggie Kebabs with Peanut-sriracha Sauce

SmartPoints value: Green plan: 7SP, Blue plan - 3SP, Purple plan - 3SP

Total Time: 41 min, Prep time: 35 min, Cooking time: 6 min, Serves: 4

Nutritional value: Calories - 144.7, Carbs - 9.5g Fat - 8.9g, Protein - 8.8g

Are you planning to go meatless at your next barbecue? Veggie kebabs are your perfect companion. These broccoli, tofu, and radish favorites offer a delicious option for a vegetarian, vegan, or someone who demands a fresher take on the usual cookout. Put the kebabs together quickly in the kitchen.

Then, brush them with an easy-to-make savory sauce before placing them on the grill. Powdered peanut butter makes this nutritious sauce that adds loads of flavor to the favorites.

Cooking them takes about six minutes, and they are perfect for your next picnic. You can pair them with a fresh side salad to increase the vegetable tally.

Ingredients

- Broccoli (uncooked) - 10 oz, florets (about 4 cups)

- Cooking spray - 4 spray(s)
- Firm tofu (rinsed and drained) - 28 oz
- Table salt - ½ tsp
- Radish(es) (fresh, trimmed and halved) - 8 medium
- Lime juice (fresh) - 1½ Tbsp
- Peanut butter (powdered) - 6 Tbsp
- Water - 4½ Tbsp
- Ketchup - 3 Tbsp
- White miso - 3 Tbsp, (low-sodium)
- Soy sauce (low-sodium) - 1½ Tbsp
- Sriracha hot sauce - 1½ tsp
- Sesame oil (toasted) - 1½ tsp
- Sesame seeds (unsalted toasted) - 1 Tbsp

Instructions

1.   Soak up to eight 10-inches bamboo skewers in a shallow dish containing water for at least 20 minutes (or use metal skewers).

2.   Put water in a large saucepan and bring it to a boil over high heat. Add salt and radishes to the pan and cook for 5 minutes.

3.   Add broccoli and cook for 1 minute more. Drain a colander into the saucepan and its content, then Dash the vegetables under

cold water until it is cool to the touch. Drain it properly; Pat it dry with paper towels.

4.   Dry out the tofu blocks with paper towels and cut each block into 12 even cubes.

5.   To prepare the sauce, stir the water and powdered peanut butter together in a medium bowl to form a smooth, loose paste.

6.   Add lime juice, ketchup, miso, Sriracha, soy sauce, and oil, then stir to mix.

7.   To prepare kebabs, thread two broccoli florets, two radish halves, and three tofu cubes on each skewer.

8.   Apply medium-high heat to a grill. Brush the kebabs with sauce on one side and lightly coat with cooking spray off the heat.

9.   Place the kebabs on the grill, sauce side down and cook for 2-3 minutes.

10.   Brush the other side with the sauce, flip it and cook for another 2-3 minutes.

11.   Remove the kebabs from the grill and brush them with extra sauce, then sprinkle them with sesame seeds before serving.

Crockpot Beef Stew

Using a crockpot for stew is not just comfortable but also guarantees that I don't burn it to the bottom of the pot. I love the fact that I can refrigerate my stew in the crockpot overnight, and the next morning, all I need to do is put it in the crockpot base and turn it on.

If you are thinking of a fitting meal for a cold winter evening, give this beef stew a try. It is one of the highly-rated meals over time. I believe the taste will leave you wanting more.

SmartPoints value: Green plan - 6SP, Blue plan - 6SP, Purple plan - 6SP

SmartPoints value: Green plan - 6SP, Blue plan - 6SP, Purple plan - 6SP

Total Time: 1hr 15min, Prep time: 15 min, Cooking time: 1hr, Serves: 8

Nutritional value: Calories – 343, Carbs – 23.5g, Fat – 17.3g, Protein – 22.2g

Ingredients

- Beef chuck roast - 2 lb

- Russet potatoes (2-in diameter) - 4 medium
- Carrots - 4 medium
- Onion - 1 large
- Garlic - 4 cloves
- Onion soup mix - 1 packet
- Fat-free beef broth - 8 cups
- Celery stalks (chopped) - 4 medium
- Add salt and pepper (to taste)

Instructions

1. Chop the roast into pieces (1 inch)

2. Cut peeled potatoes into slices (1/2 inch)

3. Cut peeled carrots into equal chunks (1/2 inch)

4. Cut onion into large pieces

5. Mix the beef, celery, carrots, potatoes, onion, garlic, onion soup mix and beef broth inside the crockpot

6. Add seasoning to taste (salt and pepper)

7. Cook till it's ready

8. This meal is easy to prepare. All you need to do is give it a try and enjoy it.

Elegant Corn Salad

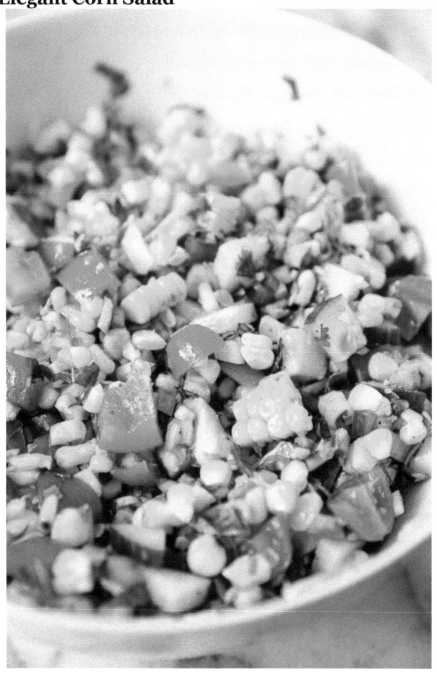

Serving: 6

Prep Time: 10 minutes

Cooking Time: 2 hours

Ingredients:

- 2 ounces prosciutto, cut into strips
- 1 teaspoon olive oil
- 2 cups corn
- 1/2 cup salt-free tomato sauce
- 1 teaspoon garlic, minced
- 1 green bell pepper, chopped

How To:

1. Grease your Slow Cooker with oil.

2. Add corn, prosciutto, garlic, tomato sauce, bell pepper to your Slow Cooker.

3. Stir and place lid.

4. Cook on HIGH for 2 hours.

5. Divide between serving platters and enjoy!

Nutrition (Per Serving)

Calories: 109

Fat: 2g

Carbohydrates: 10g

Protein: 5g

Arabic Fattoush Salad

Serving: 4

Prep Time: 15 minutes

Cook Time: 2-3 minutes

Ingredients:

- 1 whole wheat pita bread
- 1 large English cucumber, diced
- 2 cup grape tomatoes, halved
- ½ medium red onion, finely diced
- ¾ cup fresh parsley, chopped
- ¾ cup mint leaves, chopped
- 1 clove garlic, minced
- ¼ cup fat free feta cheese, crumbled
- 1 tablespoon olive oil
- 1 teaspoon ground sumac
- Juice from ½ a lemon
- Salt and pepper as needed

How To:

1. Mist pita bread with cooking spray.

2. Season with salt.

3. Toast until the breads are crispy.

4. Take a large bowl and add the remaining ingredients and mix (except feta).

5. Top the mix with diced toasted pita and feta.

6. Serve and enjoy!

Nutrition (Per Serving)

Calories: 86

Fat: 3g

Carbohydrates: 9g

Protein: 9g

Heart Warming Cauliflower Salad

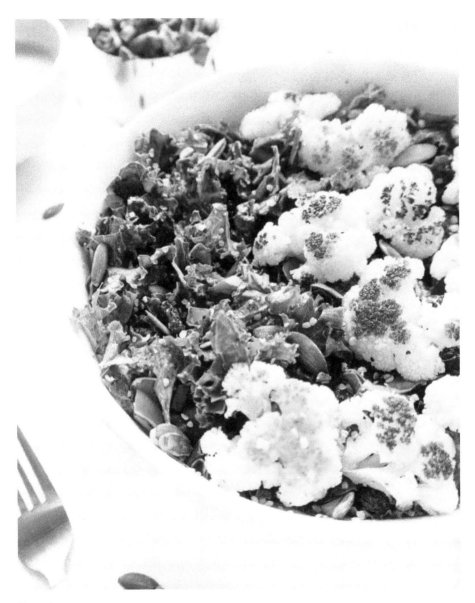

Serving: 3

Prep Time: 8 minutes

Cook Time: nil

Ingredients:

- 1 head cauliflower, broken into florets
- 1 small onion, chopped
- 1/8 cup extra virgin olive oil
- ¼ cup apple cider vinegar
- ½ teaspoon of sea salt
- ½ teaspoon of black pepper
- ¼ cup dried cranberries
- ¼ cup pumpkin seeds

How To:

1. Wash the cauliflower and break it up into small florets.

2. Transfer to a bowl.
3. Whisk oil, vinegar, salt and pepper in another bowl.
4. Add pumpkin seeds, cranberries to the bowl with dressing.
5. Mix well and pour the dressing over the cauliflower.
6. Add onions and toss.
7. Chill and serve.
8. Enjoy!

Nutrition (Per Serving)

Calories: 163

Fat: 11g

Carbohydrates: 16g

Protein: 3g

Great Greek Sardine Salad

Serving: 2

Prep Time: 10 minutes

Cook Time: 10 minutes

Ingredients:

- 2 tablespoons extra virgin olive oil
- 1 garlic clove, minced
- 2 teaspoons dried oregano
- ½ teaspoon freshly ground pepper
- 3 medium tomatoes, cut into large sized chunks
- 1 can (15 ounces) rinsed chickpeas
- 1/3 cup feta cheese, crumbled
- ¼ cup red onion, sliced
- 2 tablespoons Kalamata olives, sliced
- 2 cans 4-ounce drained sardines, with bones and packed in either oil or water

How To:

1. Take a large bowl and whisk in lemon juice, oregano, garlic, oil, pepper and mix well.

2. Add tomatoes, chickpeas, cucumber, olives, feta and mix.

3. Divide the salad amongst serving platter and top with sardines.

4. Enjoy!

Nutrition (Per Serving)

Calories: 347

Fat: 18g

Carbohydrates: 29g

Protein: 17g

Shrimp and Egg Medley

Serving: 4

Prep Time: 15 minutes

Cook Time: nil

Ingredients:

- 4 hard boiled eggs, peeled and chopped
- 1 pound cooked shrimp, peeled and deveined, chopped
- 1 sprig fresh dill, chopped
- ¼ cup mayonnaise
- 1 teaspoon Dijon mustard
- 4 fresh lettuce leaves

How To:

1. Take a large serving bowl and add the listed ingredients (except lettuce).

2. Stir well.

3. Serve over bed of lettuce leaves.

4. Enjoy!

Nutrition (Per Serving)

Calories: 292

Fat: 17g

Carbohydrates: 1.6g

Protein: 30g

Chicken breast

- 1 skinless, boneless (3 ounces)
- Diced zucchini – ½ cup
- Diced potato – ½ cup
- Diced onion – ¼ cup
- Sliced baby carrots – ¼ cup
- Sliced mushrooms – ¼ cup
- Garlic powder – 1/8 tsp.
- Italian seasoning – ¼ tsp.

Method

1.   Preheat oven to 350F.

2.   Grease a parchment paper with cooking spray.

3.   On the foil, add chicken, top mushrooms, carrots, onion, potato, and zucchini. Sprinkle with Italian seasoning and garlic powder.

4.   Fold the foil to make a packet.

5.   Place the packet on a cookie sheet.

6.   Bake until chicken and vegetables are tender, about 45 minutes.

7.   Serve.

Nutritional Facts Per Serving

Calories: 207

Fat: 2.5g

Carb: 23g

Protein: 23g

Sodium 72mg

Healthy Berry Cobbler

Serving: 8

Prep Time: 10 minutes

Cooking Time: 2 hours 30 minutes

Ingredients:

- 1 ¼ cups almond flour
- 1 cup coconut sugar
- 1 teaspoon baking powder
- ½ teaspoon cinnamon powder
- 1 whole egg
- ¼ cup low-fat milk
- 2 tablespoons olive oil
- 2 cups raspberries
- 2 cups blueberries

How To:

1.   Take a bowl and add almond flour, coconut sugar, baking powder and cinnamon.

2. Stir well .

3. Take another bowl and add egg, milk, oil, raspberries, blueberries and stir.

4. Combine both of the mixtures.

5. Grease your Slow Cooker.

6. Pour the combined mixture into your Slow Cooker and cook on HIGH for 2 hours 30 minutes.

7. Divide between serving bowls and enjoy!

Nutrition (Per Serving)

Calories: 250

Fat: 4g

Carbohydrates: 30g

Protein: 3g

Tasty Poached Apples

Serving: 8

Prep Time: 10 minutes

Cooking Time: 2 hours 30 minutes

Ingredients:

- 6 apples, cored, peeled and sliced
- 1 cup apple juice, natural
- 1 cup coconut sugar
- 1 tablespoon cinnamon powder

How To:

1. Grease Slow Cooker with cooking spray.

2. Add apples, sugar, juice, cinnamon to your Slow Cooker.
3. Stir gently.
4. Place lid and cook on HIGH for 4 hours.
5. Serve cold and enjoy!

Nutrition (Per Serving)

Calories: 180

Fat: 5g

Carbohydrates: 8g

Protein: 4g

Home Made Trail Mix For The Trip

Serving: 4

Prep Time: 10 minutes

Cook Time: 55 minutes

Ingredients:

- ¼ cup raw cashews
- ¼ cup almonds
- ¼ cup walnuts
- 1 teaspoon cinnamon
- 2 tablespoons melted coconut oil
- Sunflower seeds as needed

How To:

1. Line baking sheet with parchment paper.

2. Pre-heat your oven to 275 degrees F.

3. Melt coconut oil and keep it on the side.

4. Combine nuts to large mixing bowl and add cinnamon and melted coconut oil.

5.   Stir.

6.   Sprinkle sunflower seeds.

7.   Place in oven and brown for 6 minutes.

8.   Enjoy!

Nutrition (Per Serving)

Calories: 363

Fat: 22g

Carbohydrates: 41g

Protein: 7g

Heart Warming Cinnamon Rice Pudding

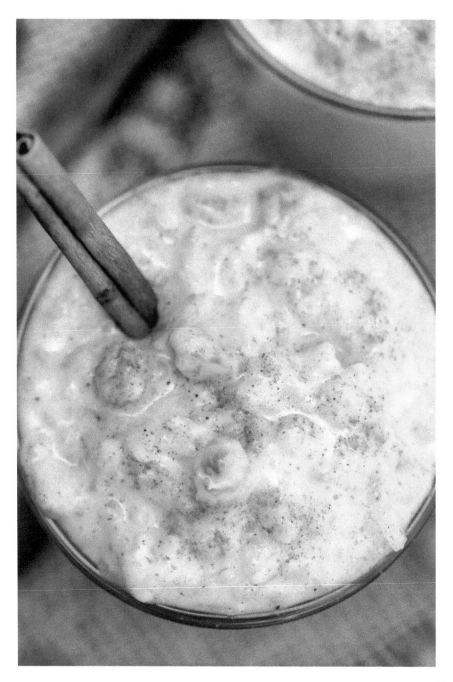

Serving: 4

Prep Time: 10 minutes

Cooking Time: 5 hours

Ingredients:

- 6 ½ cups water
- 1 cup coconut sugar
- 2 cups white rice
- 2 cinnamon sticks
- ½ cup coconut, shredded

How To:

1. Add water, rice, sugar, cinnamon and coconut to your Slow Cooker.

2. Gently stir.
3. Place lid and cook on HIGH for 5 hours.
4. Discard cinnamon.
5. Divide pudding between dessert dishes and enjoy!

Nutrition (Per Serving)

Calories: 173

Fat: 4g

Carbohydrates: 9g

Protein: 4g

Pure Avocado Pudding

Serving: 4

Prep Time: 3 hours

Cook Time: nil

Ingredients:

1 cup almond milk

- 2 avocados, peeled and pitted
- ¾ cup cocoa powder
- 1 teaspoon vanilla extract
- 2 tablespoons stevia
- ¼ teaspoon cinnamon
- Walnuts, chopped for serving

How To:

1.   Add avocados to a blender and pulse well.

2.   Add cocoa powder, almond milk, stevia, vanilla bean extract and pulse the mixture well.

3.   Pour into serving bowls and top with walnuts.

4.   Chill for 2-3 hours and serve!

Nutrition (Per Serving)

Calories: 221

Fat: 8g

Carbohydrates: 7g

Protein: 3g

Authentic Ginger and Berry Smoothie

Serving: 2

Prep Time: 5 minutes

Cook Time: Nil

Ingredients:

- 2 cups blackberries
- 2 cups unsweetened almond milk
- 1 -2 packs of stevia
- 1 piece of 1-inch fresh ginger, peeled and roughly chopped
- 2 cups crushed ice

How To:

1.   Add the listed ingredients to a blender and blend the whole mixture until smooth.

2.   Serve chilled and enjoy!

Nutrition (Per Serving)

Calories: 200

Fat: 10g

Carbohydrates: 14g

Protein 2g

A Glassful of Kale and Spinach

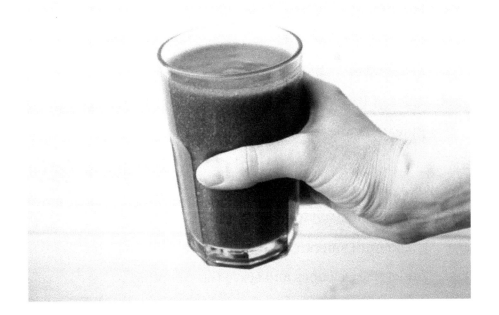

Serving: 2

Prep Time: 5 minutes

Ingredients:

- Handful of kale
- Handful of spinach
- 2 broccoli heads
- 1 tomato
- Handful of lettuce
- 1 avocado, cubed
- 1 cucumber, cubed
- Juice of ½ lemon
- Pineapple juice as needed

How To:

1. Add all the listed ingredients to your blender.
2. Blend until smooth.
3. Add a few ice cubes and serve the smoothie.
4. Enjoy!

Nutrition (Per Serving)

Calories: 200

Fat: 10g

Carbohydrates: 14g

Protein 2g

Green Tea, Turmeric, and Mango Smoothie

Serving: 2

Prep Time: 5 minutes

Ingredients:

- 2 cups mango, cubed
- 2 teaspoons turmeric powder
- 2 tablespoons Green Tea powder
- 2 cups almond milk
- 2 tablespoons honey
- 1 cup crushed ice

How To:

1.   Add the listed ingredients to a blender and blend the whole mixture until smooth.

2.   Serve chilled and enjoy!

Nutrition (Per Serving)

Calories: 200

Fat: 10g

Carbohydrates: 14g

Protein 2g

The Great Anti-Oxidant Glass

Serving: 2

Prep Time: 5 minutes

Ingredients:

- 1 whole ripe avocado
- 4 cups organic baby spinach leaves
- 1 cup filtered water
- Juice of 1 lemon
- 1 English cucumber, chopped
- 3 stems fresh parsley
- 5 stems fresh mint
- 1-inch piece fresh ginger
- 2 large ice cubes

How To:

1. Add all the listed ingredients to your blender.
2. Blend until smooth.
3. Add a few ice cubes and serve the smoothie.
4. Enjoy!

Nutrition (Per Serving)

Calories: 200

Fat: 10g

Carbohydrates: 14g

Protein 2g

Fresh Minty Smoothie

Serving: 1

Prep Time: 10 minutes

Ingredients:

- 1 stalk celery
- 2 cups water
- 2 ounces almonds
- 1 packet stevia
- 1 cup spinach
- 2 mint leaves

How To:

1. Add listed ingredients to blender.
2. Blend until you have a smooth and creamy texture.
3. Serve chilled and enjoy!

Nutrition (Per Serving)
Calories: 417

Fat: 43g

Carbohydrates: 10g

Protein: 5.5g

Refreshing Mango and Pear Smoothie

Serving: 1

Prep Time: 10 minutes

Cook Time: Nil

Ingredients:

- 1 ripe mango, cored and chopped
- ½ mango, peeled, pitted and chopped
- 1 cup kale, chopped
- ½ cup plain Greek yogurt
- 2 ice cubes

How To:

1.   Add pear, mango, yogurt, kale, and mango to a blender and puree.
2.   Add ice and blend until you have a smooth texture.
3.   Serve and enjoy!

Nutrition (Per Serving)

Calories: 293

Fat: 8g

Carbohydrates: 53g

Protein: 8g

The Hearty Garlic and Mushroom Crunch

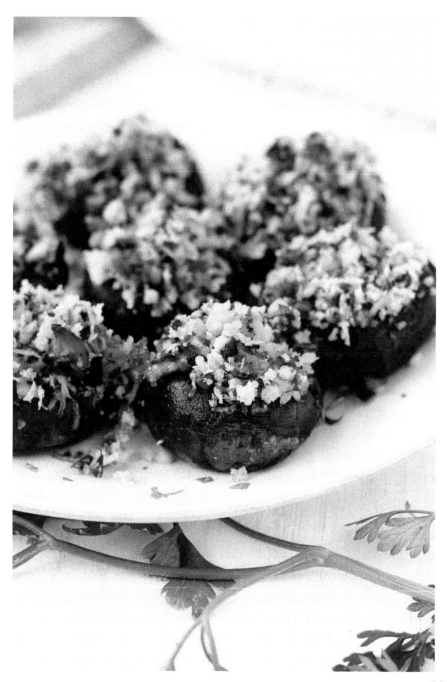

Serving: 6

Prep Time: 10 minutes

Cooking Time: 8 hours

Ingredients:

- ¼ cup vegetable stock
- 2 tablespoons extra virgin olive oil
- 1 tablespoon Dijon mustard
- 1 teaspoon dried thyme
- 1 teaspoon sea salt
- ½ teaspoon dried rosemary
- ¼ teaspoon fresh ground black pepper
- 2 pounds cremini mushrooms, cleaned
- 6 garlic cloves, minced
- ¼ cup fresh parsley, chopped

How To:

1.　　Take a small bowl and whisk in vegetable stock, mustard, olive oil, salt, thyme, pepper and rosemary.

2.　　Add mushrooms, garlic and stock mix to your Slow Cooker.

3. Close lid and cook on LOW for 8 hours.

4. Open lid and stir in parsley.

5. Serve and enjoy!

Nutrition (Per Serving)

Calories: 92

Fat: 5g

Carbohydrates: 8g

Protein: 4g

Easy Pepper Jack Cauliflower

Serving: 6

Prep Time: 10 minutes

Cooking Time: 3 hours 35 minutes

Ingredients:

- 1 head cauliflower
- ¼ cup whipping cream
- 4 ounces cream cheese
- ½ teaspoon pepper
- 1 teaspoon salt
- 2 tablespoons butter
- 4 ounces pepper jack cheese

How To:

1. Grease slow cooker and add listed ingredients.

2. Stir and place lid, cook on LOW for 3 hours.

3. Remove lid and add cheese, stir.

4.   Place lid and cook for 1 hour more.

5.   Enjoy!

Nutrition (Per Serving)

Calories: 272

Fat: 21g

Carbohydrates: 5g

Protein: 10g

The Brussels Platter

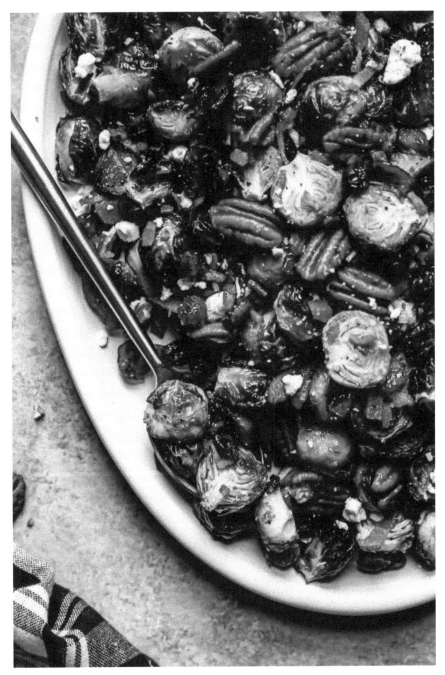

Serving: 4

Prep Time: 15 minutes

Cooking Time: 4 hours

Ingredients:

- 1 pound Brussels sprouts, bottoms trimmed and cut
- 1 tablespoon olive oil
- 1 ½ tablespoons Dijon mustard
- Salt and pepper to taste
- ½ teaspoon dried tarragon

How To:

1. Add Brussels sprouts, mustard, water, salt and pepper to your Slow Cooker

2. Add dried tarragon. 3. Stir well and cover.

3. Cook on LOW for 5 hours, making sure to keep cooking until the Brussels sprouts are tender.

4. Stir well and arrange.

5. Add Dijon over the Brussels sprouts.

6. Enjoy!

Nutrition (Per Serving)

Calories: 83

Fat: 4g

Carbohydrates: 11g

Protein: 4g

The Crazy Southern Salad

Serving: 2

Prep Time: 10 minutes

Cook Time: nil

Ingredients:

- 5 cups Romaine lettuce
- ½ cup sprouted black beans
- 1 cup cherry tomatoes, halved
- 1 avocado, diced
- ¼ cup almonds, chopped
- ½ cup of fresh cilantro
- ½ cup of Salsa Fresca

How To:

1.	Take a large sized bowl and add lettuce, tomatoes, beans, almonds, cilantro, avocado, Salsa Fresco

2.	Toss everything well and mix them

3.	Divide the salad into serving bowls and serve!

4.   Enjoy!

Nutrition (Per Serving)

Calories: 211

Fat: 16g

Carbohydrates: 6g

Protein: 10g

Kale and Carrot with Tahini Dressing

Serving: 1

Prep Time: 15 minutes

Cook Time: nil

Ingredients:

- Handful of kale
- 1 tablespoon tahnini
- ½ head lettuce
- Pinch of garlic powder
- 1 tablespoon olive oil
- Juice of ½ lime
- 1 carrot, grated

How To:

1. Add kale and roughly chopped lettuce to a bowl.

2. Add grated carrots to the greens and mix.

3. Take a small bowl and add the remaining ingredients, mix well.

4.   Pour dressing on top of greens and toss.

5.   Enjoy!

Nutrition (Per Serving)

Calories: 249

Fat: 11g

Carbohydrates: 35g

Protein: 10g

Crispy Kale

Serving: 4

Prep Time: 10 minutes

Cook Time: 25 minutes

Ingredients:

- 3 cups kale, stemmed and thoroughly washed, torn in 2-inch pieces
- 1 tablespoon extra-virgin olive oil
- ½ teaspoon chili powder
- ¼ teaspoon sea salt

How To:

1. Prepare your oven by pre-heating to 300 degrees F.

2. Line 2 baking sheets with parchment paper and keep them on the side.

3. Dry kale and transfer to a large bowl.

4. Add olive oil and toss, making sure to cover the leaves well.

5. Season kale with salt, chili powder and toss.

6. Divide kale between baking sheets and spread into single layer.

7. Bake for 25 minutes until crispy.

8. Let them cool for 5 minutes, serve.

9. Enjoy!

Nutrition (Per Serving)

Calories: 56

Fat: 4g

Carbohydrates: 5g

Protein: 2g

Cinnamon and Pumpkin Porridge Medley

Serving: 2

Prep Time: 10 minutes

Cook Time: 15 minutes

Ingredients:

- 1 cup unsweetened almond/coconut milk
- 1 cup of water
- 1 cup uncooked quinoa
- ½ cup pumpkin puree
- 1 teaspoon ground cinnamon
- 2 tablespoons ground flaxseed meal
- Juice of 1 lemon

How To:

1.   Take a pot and place it over medium-high heat.

2.   Whisk in water, almond milk and convey the combination to a boil.

3.   Stir in quinoa, cinnamon, and pumpkin.

4.   Reduce heat to low and simmer for 10 minutes until the liquid has evaporated.

5.   Remove from the warmth and stir in flaxseed meal.

6.   Transfer porridge to small bowls.

7.   Sprinkle juice and add pumpkin seeds on top.

8.   Serve and enjoy!

Nutrition (Per Serving)

Calories: 245

Fat: 1g

Carbohydrates: 59g

Protein: 4g

Quinoa and Date Bowl

Serving: 2

Prep Time: 10 minutes

Cook Time: 15 minutes

Ingredients:

- 1 date, pitted and chopped finely
- ½ cup red quinoa, dried
- 1 cup unsweetened almond milk
- 1/8 teaspoon vanilla extract
- ¼ cup fresh strawberries, hulled and sliced
- 1/8 teaspoon ground cinnamon

How To:

1.   Take a pan and place it over low heat.
2.   Add quinoa, almond milk, cinnamon, vanilla, and cook for about quarter-hour , ensuring to stay stirring from time to time.
3. Garnish with strawberries and enjoy!

Nutrition (Per Serving)

Calories: 195

Fat: 4.4g

Carbohydrates: 32g

Protein: 7g

Crispy Tofu

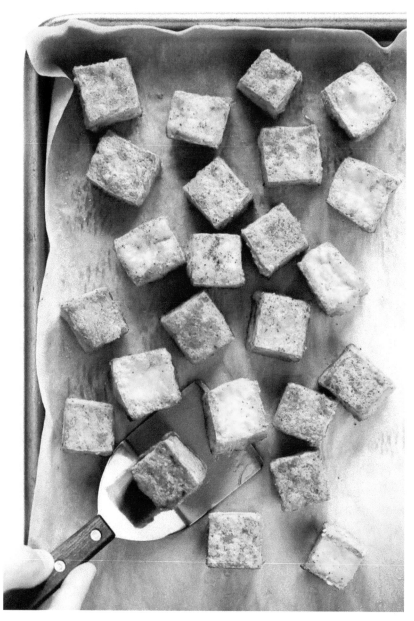

Serving: 8

Prep Time: 5 minutes

Cook Time: 20-30 minutes

Ingredients:

- 1 pound extra-firm tofu, drained and sliced
- 2 tablespoons olive oil
- 1 cup almond meal
- 1 tablespoons yeast
- ½ teaspoon onion powder
- ½ teaspoon garlic powder
- ½ teaspoon oregano

How To:

1.   Add all ingredients except tofu and vegetable oil during a shallow bowl.

2.   Mix well.

3.   Preheat your oven to 400 degrees F.

4.   during a wide bowl, add the almond meal and blend well.

5.   Brush tofu with vegetable oil , read the combination and coat well.

6.   Line a baking sheet with parchment paper.

7.   Transfer coated tofu to the baking sheet.

8.   Bake for 20-30 minutes, ensuring to flip once until golden brown.

9.   Serve and enjoy!

Nutrition (Per Serving)

Calories: 282

Fat: 20g

Carbohydrates: 9g

Protein: 12g

Hearty Pumpkin Oats

Serving: 3

Prep Time: 5 minutes

Cook Time: 8 minutes

Ingredients:

- 1 cup quick-cooking rolled oats
- ¾ cup almond milk
- ½ cup canned pumpkin puree
- ¼ teaspoon pumpkin pie spice
- 1 teaspoon ground cinnamon

How To:

1.   Take a secure microwave bowl and add oats, almond milk, and microwave on high for 1-2 minutes.

2.   Add more almond milk if needed to realize your required consistency.

3.   Cook for 30 seconds more.

4.   Stir in pumpkin puree, pie spice, ground cinnamon.

5.   Heat gently and enjoy!

Nutrition (Per Serving)

Calories: 229

Fat: 4g

Carbohydrates: 38g

Protein:10g

Wholesome Pumpkin Pie Oatmeal

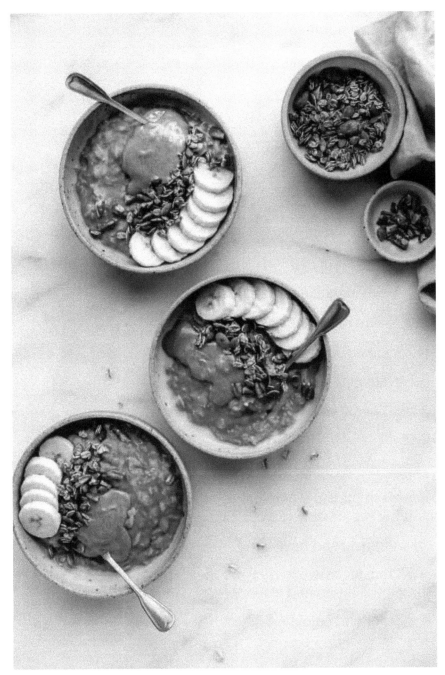

Serving: 2

Prep Time: 10 minutes

Cook Time: 10 minutes

Smart Points: 6

Ingredients:

- ½ cup canned pumpkin, low sodium
- Mashed banana as needed
- ¾ cup unsweetened almond milk
- ½ teaspoon pumpkin pie spice
- 1 cup oats

How To:

1.   Mash banana employing a fork and blend within the remaining ingredients (except oats) and blend well.

2.   Add oats and finely stir.

3.   Transfer mixture to a pot and let the oats cook until it's absorbed the liquid and is tender.

4.   Serve and enjoy!

Nutrition (Per Serving)

Calories: 264

Fat: 4g

Carbohydrates: 52g

Protein: 7g

Ulli'sGranelli

Ingredients

- 4 cups rolled oats
- 2 cups raw cashews
- 2 cups raw walnuts
- 2 cups of raw almonds
- 2 cups of fresh sunflower seed
- 2 cups of raw pumpkin seeds
- 3 cups unsweetened coconut flakes
- 1/2 cup of maple liquid syrup
- 1/4 cup of unrefined coconut oil, plus
- 2 tsp for oiling the baking sheet
- pinch of sea salt
- 1/3 cup of pure orange oil
- 2 cups of organic raisins
- 2 cups of dried cherries or cranberries

Directions

1.   Set the oven to 300°F.

2.   during a considerable bowl, mix the oats, nuts, seeds, and coconut flakes.

3.   Take alittle bowl, stir together the syrup , copra oil , salt, and orange oil till well combined, then pourover the oat-nut combination and blend nicely.

4.   Spread granola on an outsized oiled baking sheet (do it in batches if needed) and bake for 35-forty minutes untilgolden brown (rotate the baking sheet halfway via for even baking).

5.   Remove from oven and permit refreshing absolutely before mixing with raisins and dried cherries or cranberries.

6.   Store in airtight place within the fridge to stay extra crispiness.

Tofu Turmeric Scramble

Ingredients

- One 8-ounce block of firm or extra-firm tofu, drained
- 1 tbsp extra virgin olive oil
- ¼ red onion, chopped
- One green or purple bell pepper, chopped
- 2 cups of clean spinach, loosely chopped
- ½ cup sliced button mushrooms
- ½ tsp every salt and pepper
- 1 tsp garlic powder
- ½ tbsp turmeric
- ¼ cup nutritional yeast

Directions

1.   Drain the tofu and squeeze lightly to try to to away with extra water. Crumble tofu right into a bowl with the help ofhand - the smaller the pieces, the higher .

2.   Prep vegetables and region an outsized skillet at medium temperature. Once ready, then add vegetable oil , onions, and bellpeppers. Mix during a pinch of the salt and pepper and prepare dinner for about five minutes to melt the vegetables. Then add mushrooms and sauté for two mins. Then upload tofu. Sauté for about three minutes, a touch more if the tofu is watery.

3.   Add the remainder of the salt, pepper, garlic turmeric, and nutritional yeast and blend with a spatula, ensuring the spicescombo well. Cook for an additional 5 to eight mins till tofu is lightly browned.

4.   Add the spinach and canopy the pan so as to steam for 2 minutes. Serve immediately with facets of yourchoice.

5.   Nutrient CALORIES: 158

Whole Grain Cheese Pancakes

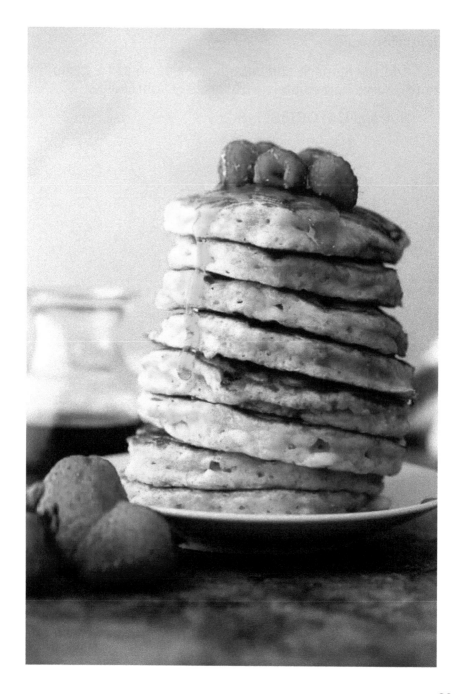

Ingredients

- 1 cup of oat flour
- 1/2 cup of sorghum flour
- 2 tbsp of teff flour
- 1/3 cup of plus 1 tbsp, tapioca starch
- 1 tbsp of baking powder
- 1/2 of tsp salt
- 3 1/2 of tsp sugar
- 1/2 tsp of flax meal
- 3/4 cup of buttermilk
- 1/3 cup of cottage cheese
- Three eggs
- half tsp vanilla extract
- 4 tsp canola oil
- 1-pint blueberries
- 1/2 cup maple syrup
- 3 tbsp water
- 1 tsp lemon juice
- pinch of salt

Instructions

1.   Combine all of your dry elements during a huge bowl and stir to combine evenly.

2.   Whisk all of your wet ingredients in another bowl collectively.

3.   Make a hole within the center of your dry substances and start to slowly pour within the wet materials, a few quartercup at a time. this may confirm that no lumps form when whisking.

4.   Continue including your wet components to the flour base till a smooth batter forms. Let the batter relax for quarter-hour at an equivalent time as you preheat your grill.

5.   While the grill is warming up, make a warm maple blueberry compote. Mix blueberries, syrup , water,lemon juice, and a pinch salt during a small pot. Stir frivolously to combine .

6.   Gently heat the pot over medium-low warmth till the blueberries start to pop and release their natural juices. Setaside, but maintain heat.

7.   Once the grill is preheated to a medium-hot temperature, lightly oil the restaurant employing a nonstick spray or asmall amount of neutral-flavored oil.

8.   Ladle the batter on to the skillet, ensuring you are doing not overload it.

9.   Give time to the pancakes to cook undisturbed until the looks of the sides dry and bubbles come to thesurface without breaking. This has got to take roughly minutes.

10.   Flip the pancakes over and cook at the opposite facet for an additional two minutes.

11.   Keep heat or serve immediately with the sweet and comfy maple-blueberry compote.

Nutrient Calories: 511

Red Pepper, Kale, and Cheddar Frittata

Ingredients

- 1 tsp olive oil

- 5 oz baby kale and spinach

- One red pepper, diced

- 1/3 cup sliced scallions

- 12 eggs

- 3/4 cup milk

- 1 cup sharp shredded cheddar cheese

- 1/4 tsp salt

- 1/4 tsp pepper

Directions

1.   Preheat oven to 375 °F .

2.   Spray an eight 1/2-inch by using 12-inch glass or casserole dish with vegetable oil or nonstick spray.

3.   Heat oil during a large frypan . Add crimson peppers on low and cook until tender. Add kale and spinach, onoccasion stirring till vegetables are wilted, or for about three min.

4.   Transfer peppers and greens to the plate, spreading evenly. Add sliced scallions.

5.   Beat eggs with milk, salt, and pepper. Pour the egg aggregate over the pan. Sprinkle cheese on top.

6.   Bake about 35-40 mins or till the mixture is totally set and starting to lightly brown. For extra color, place under broiler for an extra 1 to 3 minutes, watching to make sure the highest doesn't burn. Let cool about five mins before cutting it.

7.   Serve it as warm or refrigerate for a fast breakfast during the week

— microwave for 1-2 minutes to reheat.

Nutrient CALORIES: 77

Scrambled Eggs with Bell Pepper and Feta

Ingredients

- Olive oil-Salad or cooking-1 tsp-4.5 grams
- Green bell pepper-Sweet, green, raw-2 medium (approx 2-3/4"
- long, 2-1/2" dia)-238 grams
- Egg-Whole, fresh eggs-Four large-200 grams
- Feta cheese-1 oz-28.4 grams

Directions

1.   Heat the oil during a skillet on medium heat. Add chopped peppers and cook till tender.

2.   Stir the eggs and increase the skillet with the peppers. Stir slowly over medium-low heat till they attain your preferred doneness. Sprinkle inside the feta cheese and stir to combine and soften the cheese. Serve directly and luxuriate in it!

Nutrient

Calories 448 Carbs 14g Fat 30g Protein 31g Fiber 4g Net carbs 10g Sodium 551mg Cholesterol 769mg

Creamy Shrimp Salad

Serving: 4

Prep Time: 20 minutes

Cook Time: 5 minutes

Ingredients:

- 4 pounds large shrimp
- 1 lemon, quartered
- 3 cups celery stalks, chopped
- 1 red onion, chopped
- 2 cups mayonnaise
- 2 tablespoons white wine vinegar
- 1 teaspoon Dijon mustard
- Salt and pepper as needed

How To:

1.	Take a large pan and place it over medium heat.

2.	Add water (salted) and bring water to boil.

3.   Add shrimp and lemon, cook for 3 minutes.

4.   Let them cool.

5.   Peel and de-vein the shrimps.

6.   Take a large bowl and add cooked shrimp alongside remaining ingredients.

7.   Stir well.

8.   Serve immediately or chilled!

Nutrition (Per Serving)

Calories: 153

Fat: 5g

Carbohydrates: 8g

Protein: 19g

Passionate Quinoa and Black Bean Salad

Serving: 6

Prep Time: 5 minutes

Cook Time: 15 minutes

Ingredients:

- 1 cup uncooked quinoa
- 1 can 15 ounce black beans, drained and rinsed
- 1/3 cup cilantro, chopped
- 1 tablespoon olive oil
- 1 clove garlic, minced
- Juice from 1 lime
- Salt and pepper as needed

How To:

1. Cook quinoa according to the package instructions.

2. Transfer quinoa to a medium bowl and let it cool for 10 minutes.

3. Add remaining ingredients and toss well.

4.   Serve and enjoy!

Nutrition (Per Serving)

Calories: 188

Fat: 4g

Carbohydrates: 29g

Protein: 8g

Zucchini Noodle Salad

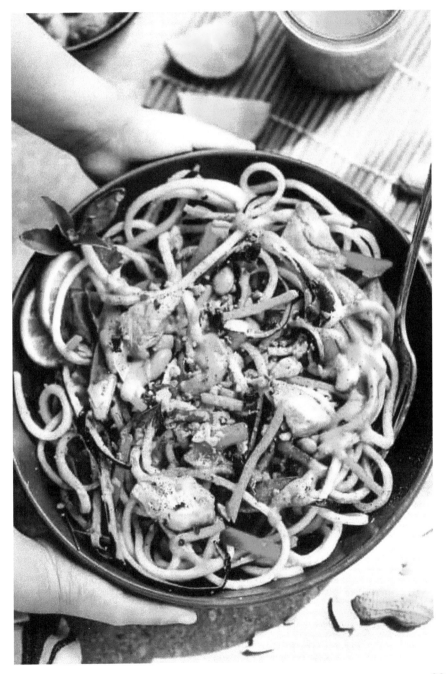

Serving: 3

Prep Time: 15 minutes

Cook Time: nil

Ingredients:

- 2 large zucchini, spiralized/peeled into thin strips
- 1 small tomato, diced
- ¼ red onion, sliced thinly
- 1 large avocado, diced
- ½ cup olive oil
- ¼ cup balsamic vinegar
- 1 garlic clove, minced
- 2 teaspoons Dijon mustard
- Salt and pepper to taste
- ¼ cup blue cheese, crumbles

How To:

1.   Take a large bowl and add zucchini noodles, onion, tomato, avocado.

2.   Take a small bowl and whisk in olive oil, vinegar, mustard, garlic, salt and pepper.

3.   Drizzle over salad and toss.

4.   Divide into serving bowls and top with blue cheese crumbles.

5.   Enjoy!

Nutrition (Per Serving)

Calories: 770

Fat: 74g

Carbohydrates: 12g

Protein: 8g

Coconut and Hazelnut Chilled Glass

Serving: 1

Prep Time: 10 minutes

Ingredients:

- ½ cup coconut almond milk
- ¼ cup hazelnuts, chopped
- 1 ½ cups water
- 1 pack stevia

How To:

1. Add listed ingredients to blender.

2. Blend until you have a smooth and creamy texture.

3. Serve chilled and enjoy!

Nutrition (Per Serving)

Calories: 457

Fat: 46g

Carbohydrates: 12g

Protein: 7g

The Mocha Shake

Serving: 1

Prep Time: 10 minutes

Ingredients:

- 1 cup whole almond milk
- 2 tablespoons cocoa powder2 packs stevia
- 1 cup brewed coffee, chilled
- 1 tablespoon coconut oil

How To:

1. Add listed ingredients to blender.

2. Blend until you have a smooth and creamy texture.

3. Serve chilled and enjoy!

Nutrition (Per Serving)

Calories: 293

Fat: 23g

Carbohydrates: 19g

Protein: 10g

Cinnamon Chiller

Serving: 1

Prep Time: 10 minutes

Ingredients:

- 1 cup unsweetened almond milk
- 2 tablespoons vanilla protein powder
- ½ teaspoon cinnamon
- ¼ teaspoon vanilla extract
- 1 tablespoon chia seeds
- 1 cup ice cubs

How To:

1. Add listed ingredients to blender.

2. Blend until you have a smooth and creamy texture.
3. Serve chilled and enjoy!

Nutrition (Per Serving)

Calories: 145

Fat: 4g

Carbohydrates: 1.6g

Protein: 0.6g

Hearty Alkaline Strawberry Summer Deluxe

Serving: 2

Prep Time: 5 minutes

Ingredients:

- ½ cup organic strawberries/blueberries
- Half a banana
- 2 cups coconut water
- ½ inch ginger
- Juice of 2 grapefruits

How To:

1. Add all the listed ingredients to your blender.

2. Blend until smooth.
3. Add a few ice cubes and serve the smoothie.
4. Enjoy!

Nutrition (Per Serving)

Calories: 200

Fat: 10g

Carbohydrates: 14g

Protein 2g

Delish Pineapple and Coconut Milk Smoothie

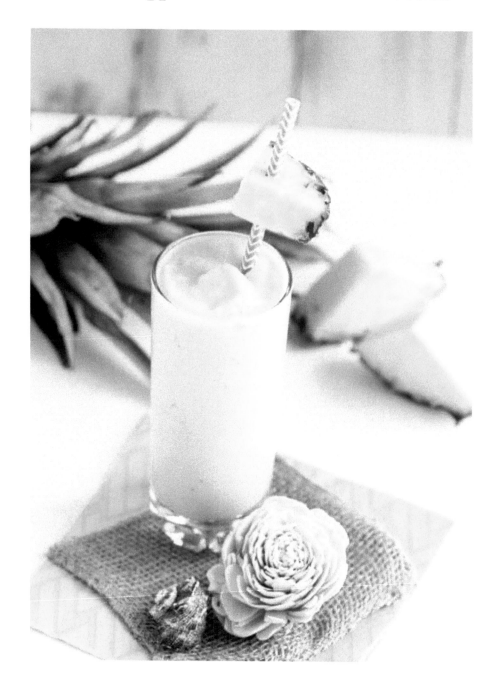

Serving: 2

Prep Time: 5 minutes

Ingredients:

- ¼ cup pineapple, frozen
- ¾ cup coconut milk

How To:

1.   Add the listed ingredients to blender and blend well on high.

2.   Once the mixture is smooth, pour smoothie in tall glass and serve.

3.   Chill and enjoy!

Nutrition (Per Serving)

Calories: 200

Fat: 10g

Carbohydrates: 14g

Protein 2g

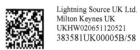

Lightning Source UK Ltd.
Milton Keynes UK
UKHW020651120521
383581UK00005B/58